PEOPLE'S REPUBLIC OF CHINA 4-MINUTE EXERCISE PLAN

(First published as Chairman Mao's 4 Minute Physical Fitness Plan)

by Maxwell L. Howell, D. Ph., Ed. D.

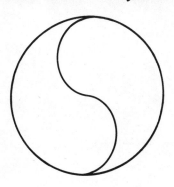

GROSSET & DUNLAP
A NATIONAL GENERAL COMPANY
PUBLISHERS • NEW YORK

First published as *Chairman Mao's 4 Minute Physical Fitness Plan* by Celestial Arts, March 1973

Grosset & Dunlap edition published August 1973

ISBN 0-448-11635-9
Published simultaneously in Canada
Printed in the United States of America

CONTENTS

INTRODUCTION 5

EXERCISE 1 . . , ... 9

EXERCISE 2 15

EXERCISE 3 21

EXERCISE 4 27

EXERCISE 5 33

EXERCISE 6 39

EXERCISE 7 45

EXERCISE 8 51

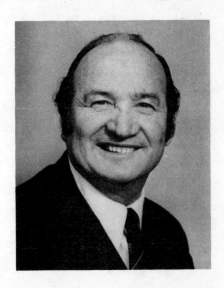

THE AUTHOR

Perhaps no one in the world is as well equipped as Dr. Max Howell to introduce these exercises to the English-speaking world. He holds two doctoral degrees, one from the University of California at Berkeley in Educational Psychology and Physical Education and the other in the History of Sport from the University of Stellenbosch, South Africa. He has approximately 200 publications and books to his credit in the history of sport, physiology of exercise, psychology of sport, and history of art and archaeology. Presently Dean of the College of Professional Studies at California State University, San Diego, he has studied and practiced sports throughout the world. In recent years he travelled three times to the USSR and once to the People's Republic of China. Dr. Howell is an ex-international rugby player, having competed for Australia, and he has been national coach of the Canadian rugby team as well as Past President of the Canadian Association of Health, Physical Education and Recreation.

PEOPLE'S REPUBLIC OF CHINA EXERCISE PLAN

The sound of a bugle came over the loudspeaker and was followed by what I later discovered were two quotations from Chairman Mao Tse-tung:
>"Promote physical culture and improve
>the people's health."
>and
>"Heighten our vigilance, defend the
>motherland."

This was followed by lively music—one . . . two . . . three . . . four . . .

My curiosity was aroused. It was my first morning in the People's Republic of China during a visit to study sport and physical education and recreation in that country. The sound of the bugle can be heard early each morning and during the work breaks at midmorning and afternoon. It signals that it is exercise time and throughout the People's Republic of China the people respond to the call. Factory workers, rural commune workers, military personnel, office workers, schoolchildren—the young and the old stop their work to do four minutes of exercise. The People's Republic of China Exercise Plan is performed.

The broadcasting day in the nation begins with these exercises so that families can perform them at home. During the day the factories stop to allow the workers to do the exercises and they are also done by the schoolchildren throughout the day. It is not uncommon to see as many as four thousand children performing the exercises together at schools.

It is interesting to have an understanding of why the people of China, without question, have faith and belief in their national exercise program. We'll go into its background and other aspects of physical education and sports in China later. First, let's look at the 4-Minute Exercise Plan.

Many values may be attributed to the 4-Minute Exercise Plan.

1. It provides one simple, systematic exercise plan that can be performed by people of any age bracket.

2. The major muscle groups of the body are all covered.

3. The exercises include some for flexibility and are performed rhythmically. (Music adds to the enjoyment but is not a necessary requirement.)

4. Although stimulating, these exercises are not too strenuous for people who are elderly or not in the best of health.

5. The program is designed to give exercise to the whole body.

6. The plan does not require the person to lie on the ground and hence can be performed in any area.

7. The exercises can be done by large and small groups or can be performed by individuals alone.

8. No equipment is necessary.

9. The time required is only four minutes.

10. The exercises are relaxing and enjoyable to perform.

11. The exercises are excellent for women. They have a high flexibility component and aim at increasing the general muscle tones of the body.

"Promote Physical Culture and Improve the People's Health" is certainly one of Chairman Mao Tse-tung's sayings. But the saying is not unique to him. Leaders of nations throughout the world have the same or similar feelings and ideas. Today, personal physical fitness is high in the interest of the majority of people. It is now an accepted fact that when one is physically fit one is more able to enjoy life.

The People's Republic of China Exercise Plan is ideally suited for people everywhere. It should not be considered a total fitness plan but it is highly recommended. It stresses flexibility and muscle tone and, on that basis alone, has a place in any fitness program. If it is combined with a progressive cardiovascular program such as running, then, additional benefits can be derived. The exercises are best done in the morning or at night and should be performed daily at least once. You can do the series as often as you like. It is not unusual to see people doing them on their own or in small groups in the parks and in the streets of China.

Let's try the 4-Minute Exercise Plan and then we can go into the history of its development later. The program is relaxed and smooth-flowing. It takes only four minutes to perform. None of the movements or exercises is difficult to do but you may feel awkward at first, until you adjust to the flow of movement and ease of performance.

A list of suggestions to help you become adept with the exercises is below. As you study the illustrations and follow the step-by-step directions, you will quickly get the feel of the movements. You'll have a sense of exhilaration and enjoyment each time you use the Exercise Plan. Relax as you exercise. The People's Republic of China 4-Minute Exercise Plan can help you.

Suggestions:

(If you purchase the accompanying record available,[*] listen to it a few times before you start, to get the cadences.)

1. Study the pictures together with the step-by-step explanations.
2. Try the movements of the exercises several times slowly, until you feel the smoothness of the flow.
3. Again look at the pictures and think about how the movements are performed.
4. Now you are ready. Prop the book up so you can see the pictures.
   Step, step, step, step . . . Exercise 1. And off you go!

---

*A record by the Central China Philharmonic Society of the music to accompany the 4-Minute Exercise Plan is available from Celestial Arts, Millbrae, California 94030.

NOTE:
It may take several attempts before you achieve the correct pace for the movements. When that is achieved you can perform the exercises whenever you desire.

THE 4-MINUTE PLAN

The program is begun by briskly stepping in place <u>32 times</u>.

There are eight exercises which are performed in a continuous flow. Total time—<u>4 minutes</u>.

Each exercise is described in <u>8 steps</u>.

Exercises One through Seven are performed <u>4 times each</u>, and Exercise Eight is performed <u>twice</u>.

The program is concluded by running in place <u>32 times</u>.

EXERCISE 1

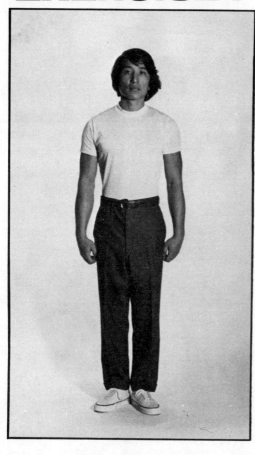

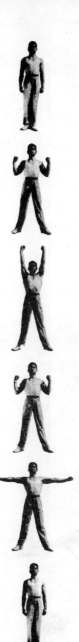

STARTING POSITION

Arms at sides, palms facing inwards. Look straight ahead, chest out, feet turned slightly outwards, heels together.

NOTE:

The program is begun by briskly stepping in place 32 times.

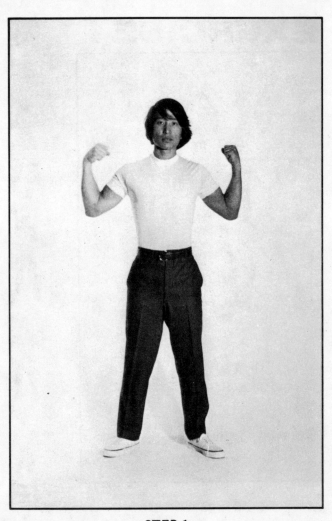

STEP 1

The left leg steps outwards; the legs are shoulder width apart. At the same time clenched fists are facing one another.

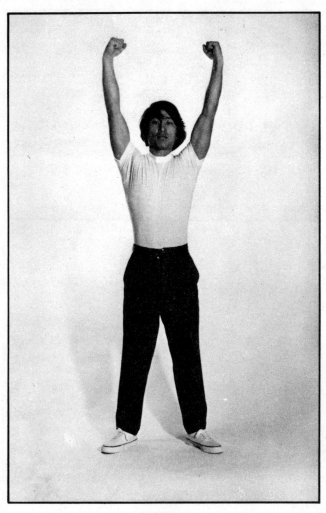

STEP 2

The arms are thrown vigorously
upwards, with the palms again
facing inwards. At the same time
the head is lifted up and the chest
is high.

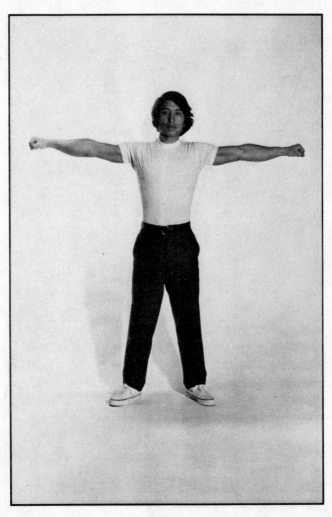

STEP 3

The arms come vigorously back
to the shoulder width position,
as in Step 1, but with the palms
facing towards the ground. The
arms are then thrown outwards,
parallel to the ground, with the
palms facing downwards.

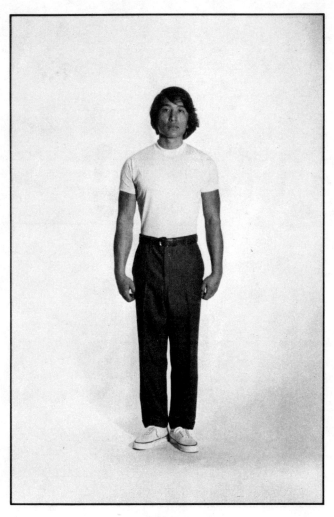

STEP 4

The left foot is drawn back and
the body returns to the starting
position.

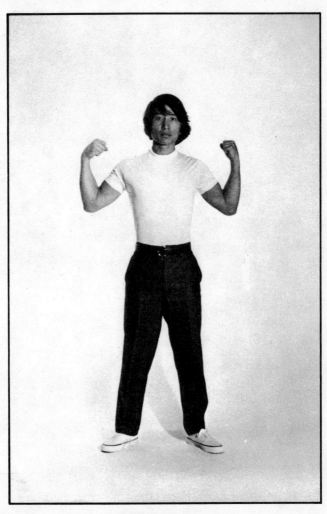

STEPS 5 to 8

Repeat Steps 1 to 4, except the right foot goes outwards. All the steps are performed vigorously.

NOTE:
This exercise is done *4 times*.

EXERCISE 2

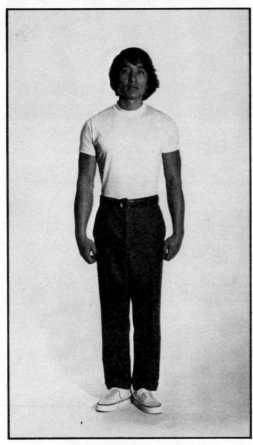

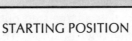

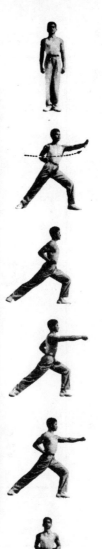

STARTING POSITION

Arms at sides, palms facing inwards. Look straight ahead, chest out, feet turned slightly outwards, heels together.

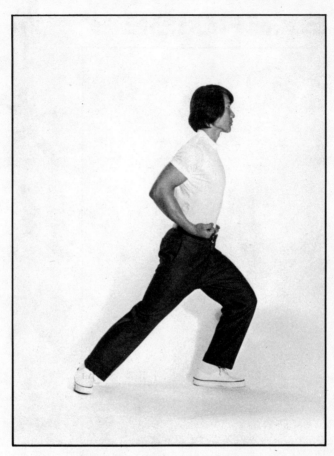

STEP 1

The left leg makes a large step outwards into the bow position. The
body turns 90° to the left. At the
same time, the open left hand
swings to the right, then straight out
over the left leg, coming to rest at
the waist in a fist. The right arm rises
to rest the fist on the waist. The
palms of both clenched fists face
upwards.

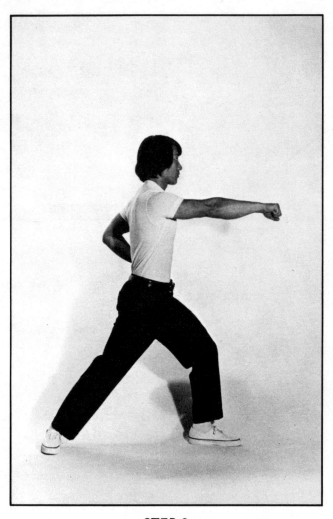

STEP 2

The right hand punches straight and the wrist rotates so the palm faces down. The arm is parallel to the ground, fist remains clenched.

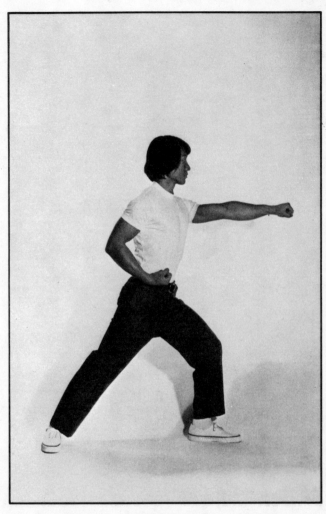

STEP 3

The left hand punches out vigorously, palm towards the ground. At the same time, the right fist returns to the waist, palm up.

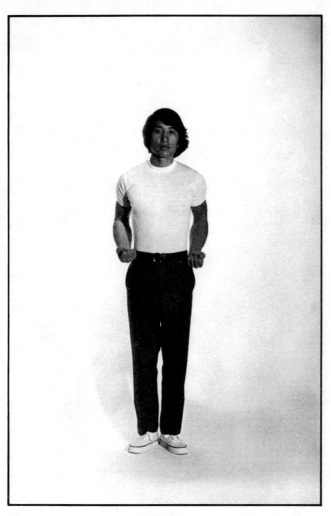

STEP 4

Bring the left foot back, turn the body to the front, bring the left fist back to the waist, palms of both fists facing up.

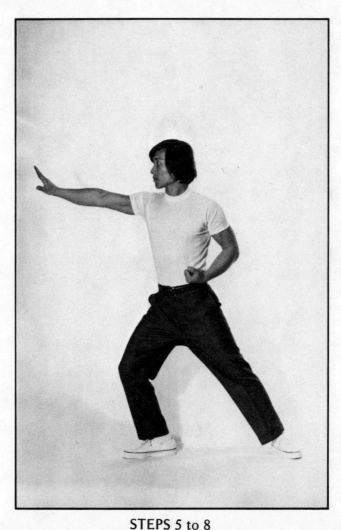

STEPS 5 to 8

Repeat Steps 1 to 4, except the right foot goes outwards. Return to the erect position.

NOTE:

This exercise is done 4 *times.*

POINTS TO REMEMBER:

When punching, the fist rotates.

EXERCISE 3

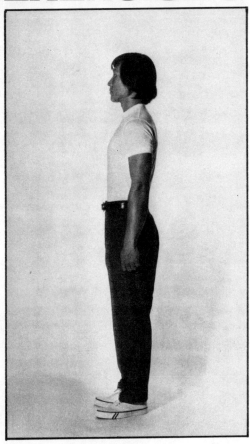

STARTING POSITION

Arms at sides, palms facing inwards. Look straight ahead, chest out, feet turned slightly outwards, heels together.

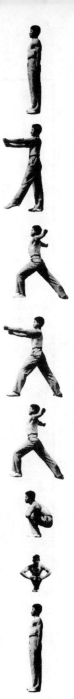

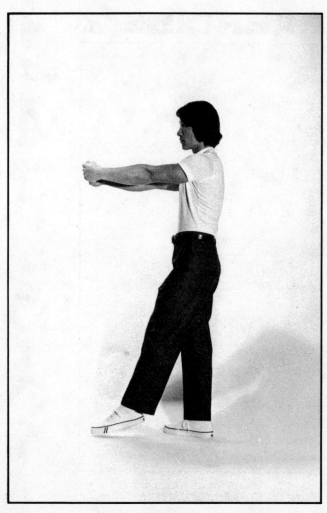

STEP 1

The left foot steps out into the
bow position. At the same time
the two hands go out towards
the front of the body and clench
together, palms facing inwards.
The arms are then stretched out
towards the back.

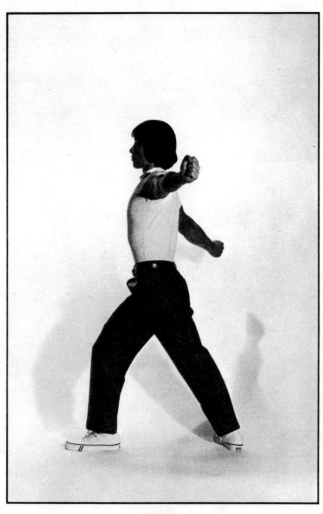

STEP 2

Step 1 is repeated with the feet in in the same position.

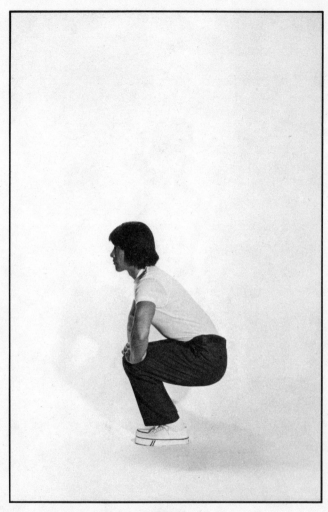

STEP 3

The left leg comes back and, as the feet come together, squat with both hands holding the knees. The fingers face each other. The elbows are out.

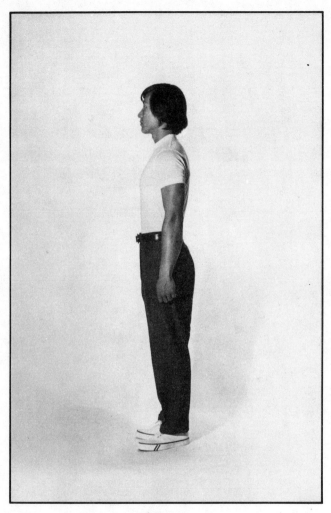

STEP 4
Return to the erect position.

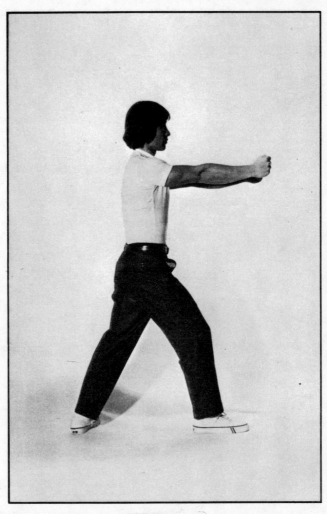

STEPS 5 to 8

Repeat Steps 1 to 4, except the right foot goes forward.

NOTE:
This exercise is done *4 times*.

POINTS TO REMEMBER:
1. Expand the chest.
2. Keep shoulders back and straight.

EXERCISE 4

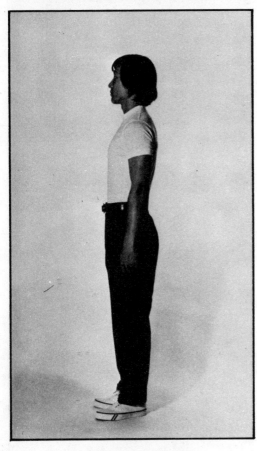

STARTING POSITION

Arms at sides, palms facing inwards. Look straight ahead, chest out, feet turned slightly outwards, heels together.

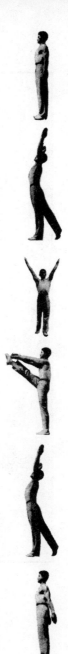

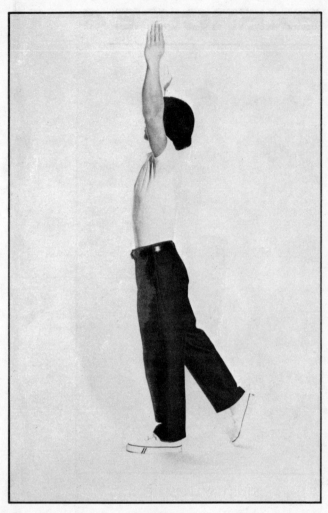

STEP 1

The right leg steps backwards, with the toe pointed and touching the ground. The weight remains on the left foot, which remains flat on the ground. At the same time the arms are thrust forward and upward, palms facing inwards, into a "V" position.

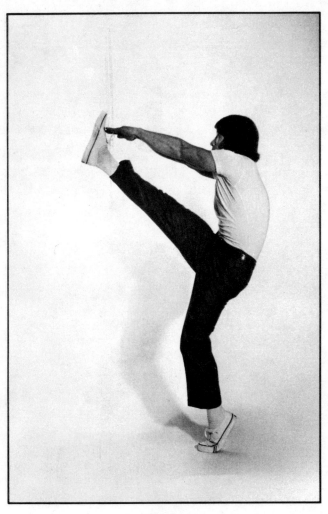

STEP 2

The right leg kicks upwards, keep-
ing straight. There is no bend of
the knee. At the same time both
hands come down to touch the
instep.

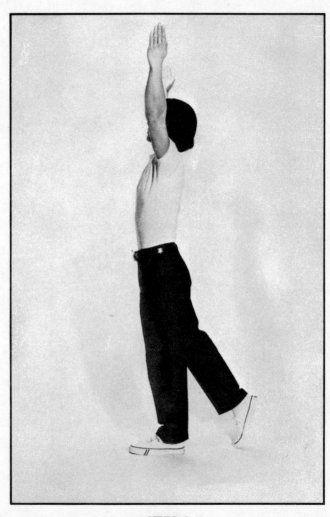

STEP 3
Return to the Step 1 position.

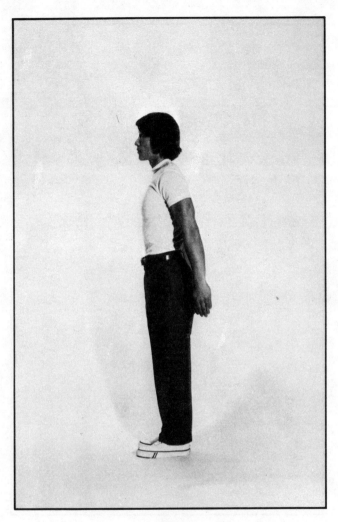

STEP 4

The right foot is brought forward. The two arms come down naturally and are swung back slightly.

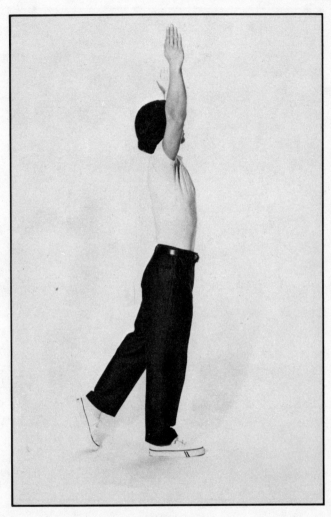

STEPS 5 to 8

Repeat Steps 1 to 4, except the left leg steps backwards. For the end of Step 8, return to the starting position.

NOTE:
This exercise is done *4 times*.

EXERCISE 5

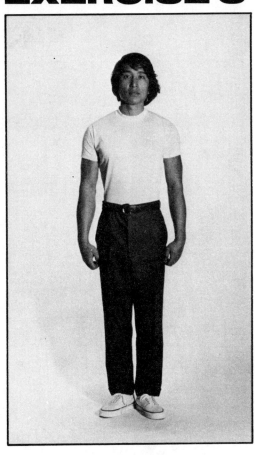

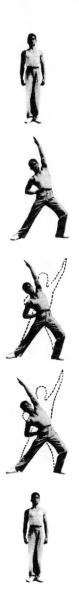

STARTING POSITION

Arms at sides, palms facing inwards. Look straight ahead, chest out, feet turned slightly outwards, heels together.

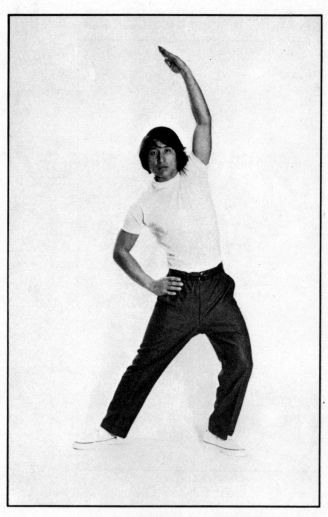

STEP 1

The left leg steps outwards, a large step, into the bow position.

At the same time the right hand goes to the waist; the left arm goes from the side to above the head, arm straight, the palm facing inwards. The whole body moves with this action and there is a slight bend to the right.

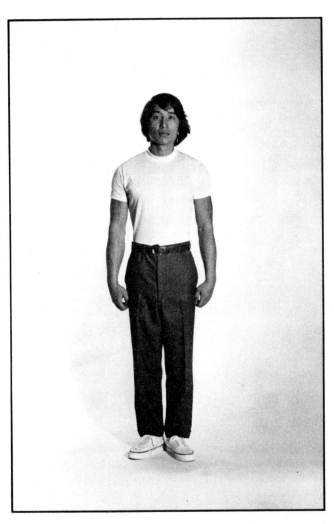

STEP 2

Return to the upright position.
Repeat the bending procedure.

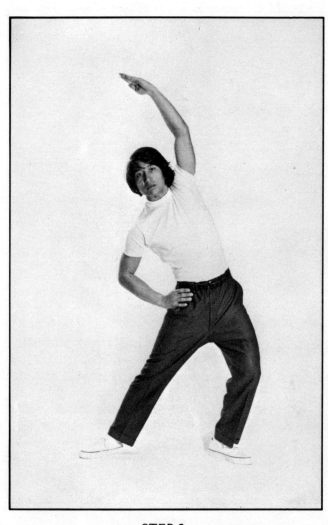

STEP 3

Return to the upright position.
Repeat the bending procedure.

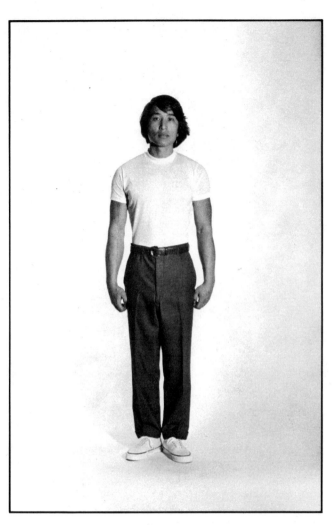

STEP 4

The left leg returns to the original position. At the same time both arms go to the sides and the body then returns to the starting position.

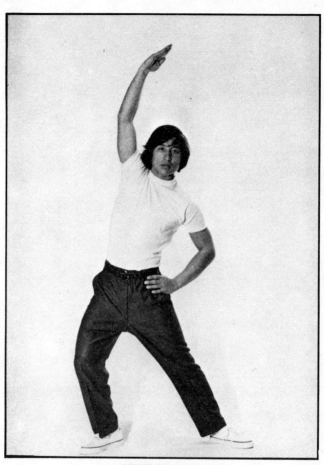

STEPS 5 to 8
Same as 1 to 4, except the right
leg steps outward and the opposite
side of the body is used.

NOTE:
This exercise is done *4 times.*

POINTS TO REMEMBER:
1. The degree of bend is increased each
   time.
2. When bending the body you should
   lower the head with your body. The
   body should not lean forward or
   turn.
3. During the second and third bend-
   ings the rhythm of the legs and
   upper body should be in unison.

EXERCISE 6

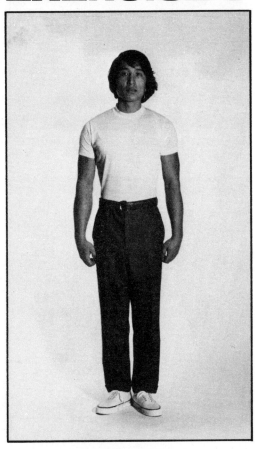

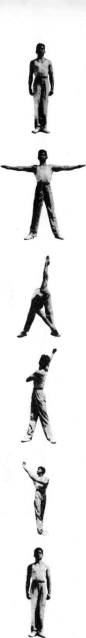

STARTING POSITION

Arms at sides, palms facing inwards. Look straight ahead, chest out, feet turned slightly outwards, heels together.

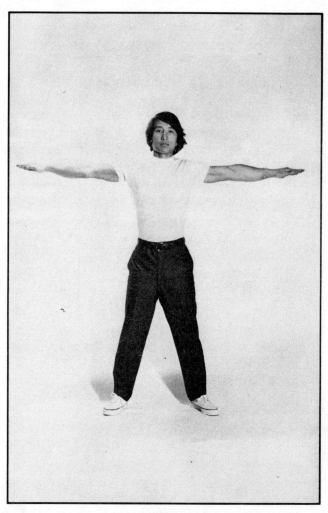

STEP 1

The left leg is extended outwards slightly, under the shoulder. At the same time both arms are extended out to the side, shoulder height, palms facing the ground.

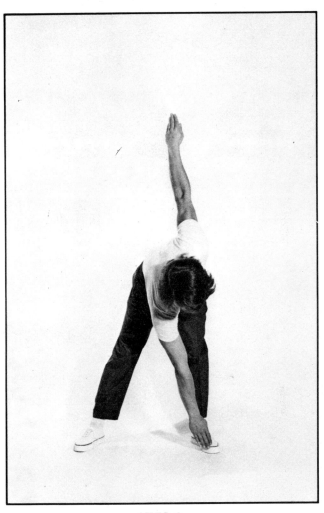

STEP 2

The right hand touches the front of the left foot, the left arm is extended high.

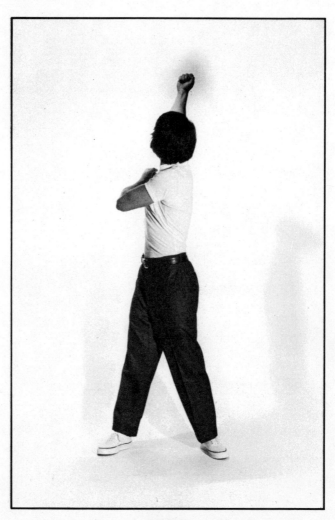

STEP 3

The upper body is raised, the fists are clenched and the body rotates towards the upper right position. The right arm extends straight out and up, the left arm bends to the front of the chest. The eyes look at the right hand.

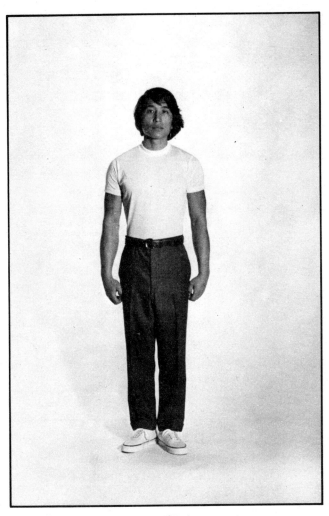

STEP 4

The left leg, the arms and the body return to the starting position.

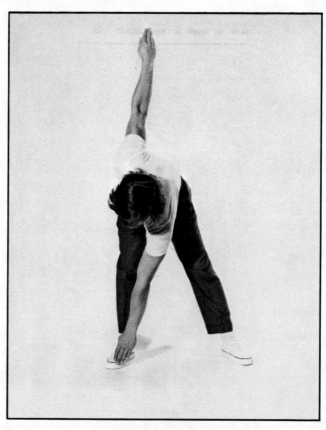

STEPS 5 to 8
Same as 1 to 4, except the right leg is extended outwards slightly and the opposite side of the body is used.

NOTE:
This exercise is done *4 times*.

POINTS TO REMEMBER:
1. When the body is rotated the legs do not move and the heels are not raised.
2. When rotating to the front the legs should be straight.

EXERCISE 7

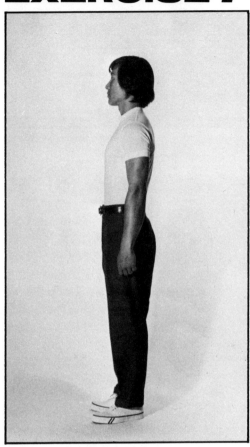

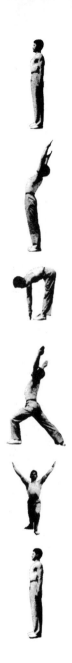

STARTING POSITION

Arms at sides, palms facing inwards. Look straight ahead, chest out, feet turned slightly outwards, heels together.

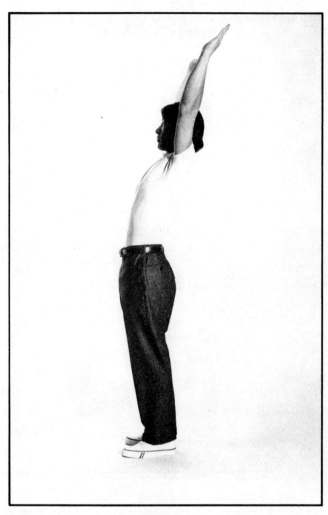

STEP 1

Both arms are raised upward, palms facing forward, and, at the same time, the upper body bends backwards.

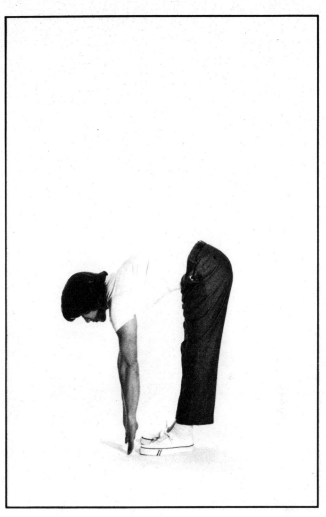

STEP 2

The upper body bends forward,
the fingers touch the ground.

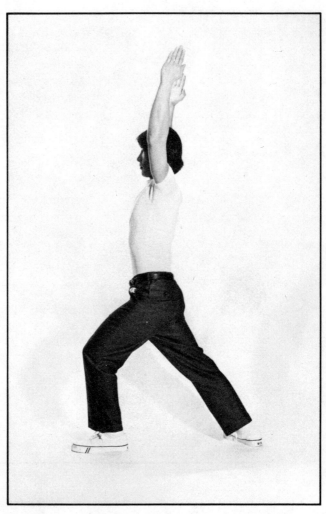

STEP 3

The body is raised, both arms are extended upward in a "V" shape position, the palms facing each other. At the same time the left leg takes one large step forward and is in the bow-shape position. The body bends backwards. The head is raised slightly.

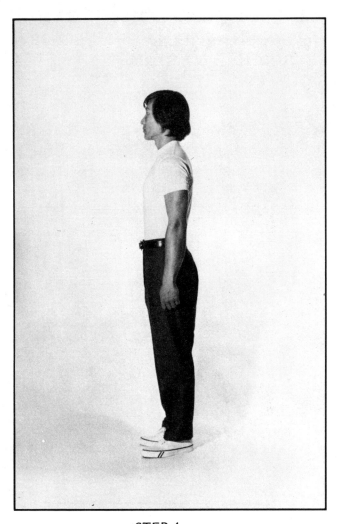

STEP 4

The left leg returns, the arms and the body return to the starting position.

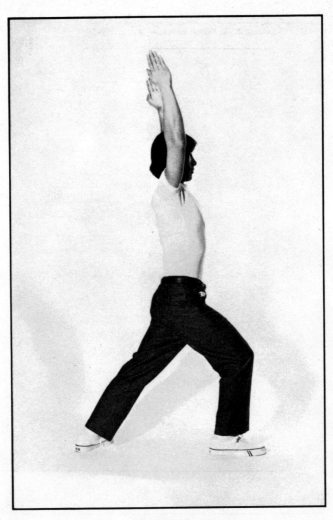

STEPS 5 to 8

The same as Steps 1 to 4, except in Step 7 the right leg goes forward.

NOTE:
This exercise is done *4 times*.

EXERCISE 8

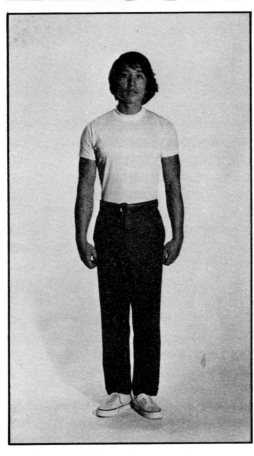

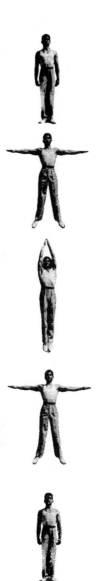

STARTING POSITION

Arms at sides, palms facing inwards. Look straight ahead, chest out, feet turned slightly outwards, heels together.

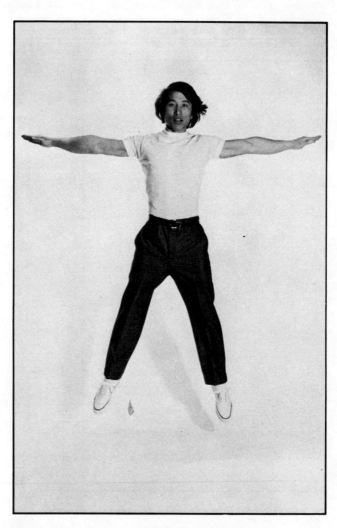

STEP 1

Jump upwards with both feet apart. At the same time both arms extend to the side at shoulder-height.

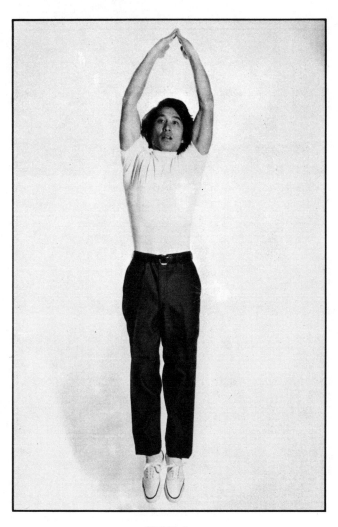

STEP 2

Jump up with the legs together.
At the same time clap the hands
above the head.

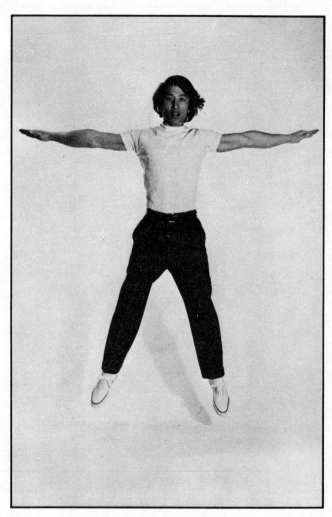

STEP 3

Repeat Step 1.

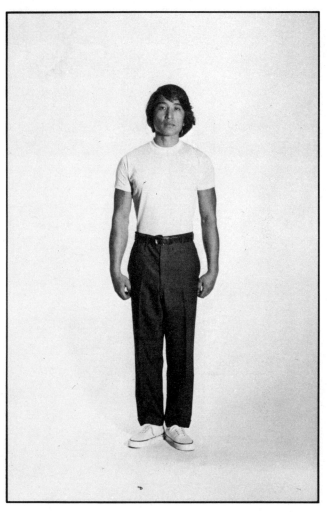

STEP 4

Jump up and bring the legs together. At the same time bring
both arms down and return to
the starting position.

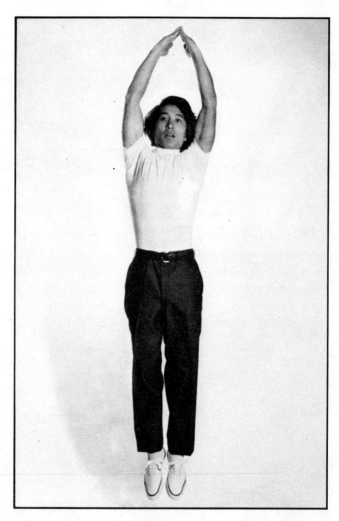

STEPS 5 to 8

As above.

NOTE:
This exercise is done *2 times*.

CONCLUSION:
The exercise program is concluded by
running in place 32 times.

The 4-Minute Exercise Plan has helped to revitalize China and can be of considerable value to people throughout the world.
Here is why.

The Role of Sport in China Today

The physical education and sports programs in the People's Republic of China are considered of primary importance. Sport occupies an integral place in Chinese Communist theory and practice. The Chinese word for physical education, **t'iyü**, when translated literally, means "bodily cultivation." Of paramount importance in life in China today is the necessity of developing and maintaining a physically fit nation.

The model for sport followed in China is basically that followed in all the Soviet bloc countries and is based on Marxist-Leninist principles. Essentially the model is the so-called triangle of sport in which the aim is mass participation and the total population, if possible, is provided with the opportunity to participate. In the U.S.S.R. one in four, say the official statistics, are members of a sports club. In addition to mass participation, the aim is to provide for sophisticated and intensive coaching for as many as possible at the local, the district, the provincial, the national and the international levels.

Each part of the triangle is considered to be important. It should be understood that some of the basic reasons for the adoption of this philosophy in the Soviet bloc and in the People's Republic of China are:

1. To improve the health of the nation thus increasing efficiency in industry and in agriculture.

2. To increase the physical culture level of the population thus ensuring the military preparation of the country.

3. To present a proper image of the country to the rest of the world through sport.

4. To keep the people occupied, boredom being the seed of revolution.

Chairman Mao's feelings and beliefs about physical education and sports.
One of Chairman Mao's earliest articles was entitled "A Study of Physical Culture." This article placed emphasis on the fact that China was weak militarily because the people of the nation were physically unfit and unable, as a result, to defend the country against its enemies. When I talked to the people in the Sports Schools and Sports Organizations in China I was unable to obtain an exact date of the writing of the article but it was between 1917 and 1923.

More important than a date of the article is a review of some of the aspects of Mao's life concerning the development of his attitude towards the importance of physical education and sports.

Mao Tse-tung studied at the Hunan Provincial Library in Changsha in 1912 and was at the First Normal School in Hunan from 1913 to 1918. It was during this period that he became interested in and concerned about physical education and sports. It was then that he came to the realization that if China were to be able to defend herself against her foes she would have to strengthen the physical fitness of each and every one of her citizens. It appears that, during these years, Mao became disillusioned with the forms of and means of physical culture and/or physical training and/or physical education which were being used in educational establishments. He also realized that, unless people were attending educational institutions, avenues of exercises were not open to the masses. He could see the degeneration of people due, in part, to lack of physical fitness, and he began to question how physically unfit people could assume responsibility and act effectively in life.

During this period he followed a rigid form of physical training and conditioning. He developed for himself a series of exercises which he performed each morning and evening. As his original, personal plan of exercises was explained to me I was interested to observe that they were very calm and mild in nature in spite of his interest in building tough, strong bodies and his interest in developing stamina. The exercises were designed to loosen the body and perhaps stimulate the flow of blood. I understand that they were a set of exercises planned to enliven and awaken the body system and muscles and to give over-all body tone.

That original exercise plan included only six exercises:

1. arm exercises—in a sitting position raising the arms in different ways and stretching.
2. leg exercises—in a sitting position raising and lowering the legs in different ways.
3. body exercises—in the standing position bending and turning the trunk.
4. head exercises—in a sitting position rotating the head.
5. slapping the body to stimulate blood flow.
6. balance exercises—in a sitting position rotating the head.

(NOTE: The present 4-Minute Exercise Plan was developed, after a number of changes through the years, by the Physical Culture and Sports Commission of the People's Republic of China.)

At that same time, Mao became a believer in cold baths to awaken the senses and almost all year round he enjoyed swimming in the waters of the Hsiang River. He also liked the rugged outdoor life of camping, hiking and mountain climbing. Perhaps these experiences helped in the Long March of 1934—35. And, also, these combined experiences doubtless influenced Mao's attitudes towards the importance of physical fitness for his then-newly-developing People's Republic of China.

So it must be realized that Chairman Mao Tse-tung's feelings in regard to physical fitness and physical education and sports are an important key to the role these activities play in life in China today.

We should also understand that, if there is a form of religion in China today, it is an infinite belief in Chairman Mao. Religion could be called the worship of Mao and his accomplishments for China and his beliefs in what the Chinese people should and must do to improve themselves and the nation.

Mao came to a realization that people had to understand the significance physical fitness played in the entirety of a person's life. He came to understand that in order to remould his nation he had to remould the thinking of people towards their own personal fitness. Only in that way could the people of China develop a personal consciousness and a belief that physical fitness makes one more able to perform all other duties in life well. If all duties of each individual are performed well, then a healthy society and nation are the end result. Chairman Mao recognized that people needed to understand the significance, in their own lives, of physical fitness so that they would participate enthusiastically in programs of exercise to increase fitness.

To achieve this outlook towards life and living, the established physical educational patterns of China had to be changed. Physical fitness had to be established as a first priority in life. People had to be taught that without a strong body life was nothing and meaningless. With a strong body an individual was more able to perform and attain other goals in life. And, to Chairman Mao, physical fitness went hand in hand with strength-of-will. The more fit a person became the greater his strength-of-will. The greater the strength-of-will of each person, the greater the nation.

Mao realized that established and acquired habits and patterns of life are hard to break and that changes in the physical activities of people would have to be introduced in a slow-flowing pattern. He also knew that an attitude had been culturally developed whereby people were ashamed to be seen exercising and would be embarrassed if seen in any form of exercise. Exercise was allied with labor. Only a peasant labored. Exercise was considered demeaning.

So, the whole attitude to life and physical fitness had to be very slowly changed. Slowly, because Mao believed that only slow change can become sure and established change. But these changes came about and today in the People's Republic of China sports and physical education are held in high esteem. It would be interesting now to briefly examine some of the avenues where the importance of physical exercise is stressed.

School physical education and sport

Physical education is considered on a par with all other subjects in the school curriculum and a well-conducted physical education program is looked upon as an important contributing factor to a healthy student body.

Two class hours of physical education a week are required and these two hour segments may be split up or given together. At the same time each student is required to do two classes of spare time activities which include extra-curricular sports activity. In addition there are special teams that train six hours per week for inter-school competition in such activities as basketball, baseball, table tennis, soccer, swimming, gymnastics and track and field. These sports are for both boys and girls with the exception of soccer. Selection to play on a school team depends on scholastic and political work as well as athletic ability.

All schools conduct mass exercises as well and the 4-Minute Exercise Plan is used.

The physical education teacher is required to demonstrate to the children the importance of physical education in life generally. The importance of physical fitness for the defense of the nation is stressed. Group awareness and mutual aid are emphasized in their team games.

Sports Schools

As well as the after-school sport a child has the opportunity of attending a Sport School. This is done at the local, the district and even at the provincial level. It is possible, at the provincial level, for a student to solely attend a Sport School where he may concentrate on a single sport in which he excels and shows expertise and take his academic classes as well. These Sports Schools are for students with exceptional athletic ability. The more normal Sports

Schools operate two or three days each week after school with superior coaches and a child elects to be coached in a particular sport.

The Chinese Sports Schools are not, at this moment, as advanced as those in the U.S.S.R. and many other Communist bloc countries, but they are moving very rapidly to try to make these programs available to as many of the school population as possible. It is a colossal project. The Russians call the sports schools their "Olympic Reserve."

The children basically use the same facilities as the competitive athlete uses and such Sports Schools can be seen in the areas which enclose gigantic sports complexes including track and field areas, swimming areas, volleyball, table tennis, gymnastics, basketball, badminton, and so on.

Sports for the adults

Again, China has not advanced to the point where, as in the U.S.S.R., one in four of the population is a member of a sports club but, through increased propaganda for the value of sport and increased coaching for the young, the Chinese public's habits and attitudes with respect to sport are being modified. As a consequence more and more adults are engaging in sport and outstanding prospects virtually become state amateurs working all year on their particular sport. They may hold jobs as well but there is little doubt that their main aim is to become a superior athlete. Some excellent facilities and outstanding coaches are available for such prospects and these are being expanded continuously.

Mass participation in sport activities is constantly encouraged. It is not uncommon for the factories to close for an hour between change-of-shifts for the workers to engage in forms of physical activity. Tug-of-war is a popular thing and large groups (both men and women together) can be seen straining on ropes in the factory grounds. Running, cycling, badminton, basketball and volleyball are also popular with factory workers.

In the rural communes time is set aside each day for sports activities of a similar nature. Different communes arrange to compete against each other in various team sports. Basketball is very popular and barefooted teams can be seen playing the game throughout the rural areas.

When one walks through the streets and parks of the large cities such as Shanghai, demonstrations of physical activities are seen with crowds gathered around to watch. It is a method of encouraging greater mass participation in physical activities. On one corner you might see Chinese Wand Drills being performed: on the next, balancing and gymnastics activities, or on the next, Chinese boxing.

Sportsmanship

One of the outstanding things to observe in the People's Republic of China is the high degree of sportsmanship. Whenever teams come together to play they stand in line facing each other and say:

"Friendship first, competition second."

Then each team, in turn, repeats:

"We learn from you."

And, before the game begins, the opposing players shake hands with each other. When any infringement of rules occurs the players involved apologize and again shake hands. Co-operation and sportsmanship are highly emphasized.

It can be seen, then, that great emphasis is placed on the importance of sports and physical activities in the life of the People's Republic of China. The need for healthy, physically-fit people in all forms of industry and agriculture is emphasized. The need of strong and healthy people who are ready and able to defend the nation is also stressed. Efforts are being made to encourage greater mass participation in all forms of sport.

And, in the every-day lives of all — young and old alike — the 4-Minute Exercise Plan is of major importance.